What is the Paleo Diet?

Your complete Paleo resource with the latest information, proper meal plans, and tips.

By Caroline G.Hawley

Legal & Disclaimer

Legal & Disclaimer

The information contained in this book is not designed to replace or take the place of any form of medicine or professional medical advice. The information in this book has been provided for educational and entertainment purposes only.

The information contained in this book has been compiled from sources deemed reliable, and it is accurate to the best of the author's knowledge; however, the author cannot guarantee its accuracy and validity and cannot be held liable for any errors or omissions. Changes are periodically made to this book. You must consult your doctor or get professional medical advice before using any of the suggested remedies, techniques, or information in this book.

Upon using the information contained in this book, you agree to hold harmless the author from and against any damages, costs, and expenses, including any legal fees potentially resulting from the application of any of the information provided by this guide. This disclaimer applies to any damages or injury caused by the use and application, whether directly or indirectly, of any advice or information presented, whether for breach of contract, tort, negligence, personal injury, criminal intent, or under any other cause of action.

You agree to accept all risks of using the information presented inside this book. You need to consult a professional medical practitioner in order to ensure you are both able and healthy enough to participate in this program.

TABLE OF CONTENTS

Introduction

The Paleo diet is the healthiest way you can eat because it is the only nutritional methodology that works with your genetics to help you stay active, and lively.

Research in science, natural chemistry, ophthalmology, dermatology and numerous other controls demonstrates that it is our advanced diet, brimming with refined foods, trans fats and sugar – all of which culminates to cause degenerative sicknesses; for example, corpulence, diabetes, coronary illness, Parkinson's, Alzheimer's, etc.

It's no wonder this diet has been gaining an increasing amount of attention in the past few years, due to its healthy effects on physical and mental health, with proper statistical data to prove it.

Here's the catch: The Paleo diet is not only based on the mainstream idea of dieting for weight loss, but it is a perfect and healthy diet for people of all ages and genders. Being on the Paleo diet removes almost all health problems from the equation, as the health problems mentioned previously were not known to be present in ancient times when people naturally ate the Paleo diet.

This eBook discusses everything you'd ever wish to know about the Paleo diet, from its crude basics and weird myths, to kick-ass recipes and weekly menus. This eBook also contains a bonus chapter on drinks that work fantastically with Paleo! What's more? Find out for yourself.

Section A: Overview

Chapter 1: What is Paleo?

The Paleo Diet — otherwise called the Stone Age, Caveman or Ancient Diet — is a current endeavor to replicate the diet of people of the Paleolithic age. These old hunter-gatherers lived before the advent of farming and subsisted on incline proteins (like fish, venison and poultry), eggs, natural products, vegetables, nuts and roots.

History

In spite of the fact that the Paleo Diet appears to be new, it has really been around for quite a few years. It was begun around the **1970s** by gastroenterologist **Walter Voegtlin** with the thought that Paleolithic precursors, who lived in a scope of time from 2.5 million to 10,000 years ago, could show present day men how to practice good eating habits.

In 2012, the Paleolithic Diet was portrayed as being one of the "most recent patterns" in diets, in light of the prevalence of diet books about it; in 2013 the diet was Google's most searched weight reduction strategy. The diet tops the list of famous modern diets globally, and draws on an appeal to nature and a narrative of conspiracy theories about how nutritional research, which does not support the gathered advantages of the Paleo Diet, is controlled by a defamed food industry.

General Nutritional Outline of the Diet

The general outline of the diet plan is as follows:

More Protein and Meat

Meat, seafood, and other creature items speak to the staple foods of cutting edge Paleo diets, since promoters claim protein constituted 19–35% of the calories in hunter- gatherer diets.

Less Carbs

In other words, non-starchy vegetables. The diet suggests the utilization of non-starchy, crisp foods grown from the ground to provide 40–48% of the daily calories and to be the primary wellspring of starches. According to the **United States Department of Agriculture, the adequate macronutrient circulation range for sugars is 48 to 68 % of aggregate calories**. An average cutting edge diet, for the most part, gets sugars from grains and dairy items, yet both of these are rejected in the Paleo diet.

More Fats

Experts prescribe that Paleo diet followers should have a moderate to higher fat allowance, as opposed to contemporary diets. The fat allowance should be comprised mainly of monounsaturated, polyunsaturated, and omega-3 unsaturated fats, and should keep away from trans fats, and Omega-6 unsaturated fats.

More Fiber

High fiber consumption is an important constituent of the Paleo Diet. This is not achieved from grains, but rather from non-starchy vegetables and natural products.

Why Opt for the Paleo Diet?

There are a great variety of physical and mental reasons why paleo is a better diet than all other fad diets, especially considering the positive health effects of paleo. Some of the main reasons why you should opt for the paleo diet are:

- Weight loss for those who are on a weight loss campaign
- Better health even though there is less restriction on calorie intake
- Diminishes the chance of many health associated medical problems like cardiac diseases, dementia, etc.
- Includes eating a lot of tasty foods during meals and snacks
- Better and healthier choices of food items including fish, eggs, meat etc.
- Keeps you away from prepackaged foods that have large amounts of chemicals and additives
- Easy to prepare meals
- Much cheaper than all other diet plans

Should You Go for Paleo?

There are numerous reasons why you might want to switch to Paleo. But if you still have questions in your mind, the following answers will help you decide if Paleo is right for you!

- Is Paleo an all protein diet? - **NO**
- Will Paleo deprive me completely of carbohydrates? – **NO, but it will restrict you to eating healthy carbs only.**
- I need to lose weight. Is Paleo safe for me? – **Yes**
- I am a vegetarian. Should I go for Paleo? – **Yes, Paleo is for all, both vegetarians and carnivores.**
- I like to have diary more. What should I do? – **Restrict your diary intake and choose natural food products.**

- What meat is recommended in Paleo? – **Most all meats are Paleo-friendly. However, stay away from highly processed meats, such as spam and hot dogs.**

- I have high blood sugar levels. Is Paleo better for me? – **Yes indeed, Paleo is the best diet for diabetic patients.**

Summing It Up

Here's the thing to remember: We're not attempting to unequivocally replicate mountain men diets. Yes, a couple of Paleo stalwarts might approach the diet this way. However, there isn't one complete, set, one-size-fits-all "Paleo diet." Some Paleo eaters go super-low-carb, while others are glad to munch on a prepared potato or a dish of white rice from time to time.

The Paleo way is sufficiently inclusive enough to fit a large variety of methodologies, however the core fundamentals of genealogical eating are still present:

- ✓ Eat whole foods that are naturally rich in vitamins and minerals. Seek out grass-fed meats, organic eggs and vegetables, and wild seafood. Enjoy nuts and seeds in moderation.

- ✓ Maintain a strategic distance from foods that will hurt you by causing systemic irritation, destroying your gut, or wrecking your common metabolic procedures. Keep away from harmful, provocative foods like gluten-containing grains, vegetables, and sugars.

Doctors, biochemists, nutritionists, and various researchers are beginning to come around to the idea of genealogical sustenance. Likewise, individuals who embrace a Paleo-style of eating are reporting significant enhancements in their general well-being and energy levels. In particular, there's proof that people who have chosen the Paleo way of eating are diminishing their dangers of various illnesses and concerns that are connected with the standard diet.

Currently about <u>25 to 30 million people around the world</u> are "Paleo" because of the healthy lifestyle it offers, keeping them away from certain degenerative diseases.

Chapter 2: Paleo Myths

Many myths are drifting around about Paleo. Despite the fact that eating Paleo is likely the healthiest diet on earth, individuals just aren't accustomed to eating that way. Shying away from great sustenance might appear to be senseless; however, like anything new and different, it requires some investment to really see its positive effects in your life.

These myths reflect the most unknown principles of Paleo cooking and eating. Let's bust them before diving further into more Paleo details!

1. Paleo is a 'fad diet'

By and large, fad diets are fleeting weight reduction plans that set unique traps and gimmicks to mask how they truly function: an amazing decrease in calorie consumption.

Fad diets are clearly designed for the short term: Extreme restriction of calories or food choices **[e.g. the 2-4-6-8 diet** (A type of diet for weight loss), in which you eat 200 calories the first day, then 400, then 600, then 800, and then cycle back to 200 and start over].

If Paleo is a fad, it must be the longest running fad ever. The truth of the matter is, people ate a Paleo diet for, by far, most of our developmental history.

With the onset of farming, people began eating grains, vegetables, dairy and liquor in significant amounts. What's more, it's just in the most recent decades that the mechanical processing of foods, and the utilization of prepared and refined foods like sugar, flour and modern seed oils became typical. Yet today, more than 70% of calories devoured in the normal diet come from these agrarian and mechanical foods. If anything is a fad, it's our current diet!

In truth, Paleo is a supplement rich, plant-based, scientifically legitimate, time-tested, and safe way to receive proper nourishment.

Maybe most critical, it conveys incredible results to those hoping to get thinner, feel better, counteract and even turn around sickness. <u>This might clarify why it was the most Googled diet in 2013, notwithstanding relentless—yet misleading—reactions by the media and restorative foundation. The facts speak for themselves.</u>

2. Paleo is low-carb

Paleo is normally lower in carbohydrates, as supplement rich foods regularly are by nature. Paleo concentrates on supplement richness, equalization, and food quality, and additionally gaining a consciousness of how food influences your body. The center isn't and never has been on carbohydrates.

The regulation of grains on a Paleo diet rapidly and effectively decreases your total carb consumption (in spite of the fact that it's essential to remember that not all Paleo diets should be low-carb, especially in athletes). Being on the Paleo diet does not mean you will be deprived of the essential carbohydrates that your body requires, but it will keep you away from carbs that can have a bad influence on your body.

3. Paleo is an all-protein diet

Protein toxicity is a real issue brought about by the measure of protein in your diet and the ratio of protein to the carbs and fats in your diet. Eating an excessive amount of protein can put weight on your kidneys and liver since they battle to break down protein.

Paleo is not a high-protein diet. Eating a variety of proteins as a part of a well-balanced diet will keep you inside of a solid scope of protein. Nowhere in a well-arranged Paleo diet do you discover a proposal to eat huge amounts of protein throughout the day; it's basically not the Paleo way.

Meat is the most basic prehistoric food, and if you eat it together with various macronutrients (starch and fat) in proper portions, your body can deal with it just fine. **A sound Paleo protein serving size is about the size of the palm of your hand, or 3 to 4 ounces for ladies and 5 to 6 ounces for men.**

4. Paleo is too expensive

If you're accustomed to buying nutritionally void, super-sized junk, then yes, Paleo will cost somewhat more. But spending wisely on your diet is much better than paying costly healthcare bills for unwanted ailments.

Here are five feasible approaches to cut down on the cost of healthy foods:

➢ **Make educated produce decisions** - Read up on the Environmental Working Group's Dirty Dozen and Clean 15 (refers respectively to the fruits and vegetables that are most and least contaminated by pesticide use)). You can utilize this data to make informed choices about the produce you buy..

➢ **Buy Locally** - Produce more often than not costs less at local produce stands and nearby farms.

➢ **Participate in a "Cow Share"** - Go to a butcher shop with companions or relatives to split the cost of beef. It's an awesome approach to get amazing meats at a lower price.

➢ **Buy in bulk** - The big-box retailers can often provide superb foods. Bring home more and save money by buying in bulk.

➢ **Stock up on deals** – Keep an eye out for sales to buy produce and the best cuts of meat at a bargain and stock up.

Chapter 3: Paleo basics

Paleo isn't about eating what you can endure. Without a doubt, a few individuals can endure grains, vegetables, dairy, and other "awful" foods, yet that is not Paleo. Paleo is about eating just naturally amazing good and tasty foods.

There are basic rules that you will have to follow when you are on the Paleo diet plan, and this chapter will clearly show you some limitations/restrictions and possible alternatives in that regard. Let's first see what to eat and what not to eat, and then we'll jump into some great Paleo recipes.

Basic Rules for Paleo

Eat a lot of meat, including beef, sheep, poultry, pork, organ meat, fish and seafood

Meat is the best source of complete protein, and eating enough protein and fat are the answer to your weight loss problems. A wide variety of meats should be on your Paleo shopping list.

Eat numerous eggs, particularly egg yolks

Try not to stress over the soaked fat myth, we will clarify that later. Eggs are particularly critical for veggie lovers who need to gain muscle and lose fat.

Eat heaps of vegetables

Here's a few: broccoli, cauliflower, finger peppers, brussel sprouts, carrots, bok choy, tomatoes, cucumbers, watercress, spinach, kale, yellow squash, zucchini, beets, turnips, parsnips... just to give some examples. Sauté them, cook them, prepare them, steam them, or broil them in coconut oil or in an Indian curry—it doesn't make a difference. Broccoli and spinach are in the main 5 superfoods and should always be on your shopping list.

Eat healthy fats

For example, animal fat (fat, tallow, bacon fat), ghee, olive oil for plates of mixed greens, coconut oil for cooking. Avocados, macadamias, almonds, hazelnuts and cashews are additionally great sources of solid fats.

Choose quality meat when looking for a healthy staple food

When buying meat, make sure you only buy lean cuts that are as fat-free as possible, as the toxins and cholesterol tend to concentrate in animal fat areas. If you're a fan of high-fat animal meat, then at least ensure that you buy only 100% grass-fed animal's meat, rather than the usual poultry or farm meat.

Go simple on bland vegetables

If your objective is fat loss, your diet should include bland vegetables such as sweet potatoes.

Keep away from grains

Grains are the main cause of various health problems due to carb over-utilization. Remove all grains from your diet: grain, wheat, corn, oats, rice, etc.

Keep away from sugar

Keep away from all types of sugar, not simply table sugar. That includes syrups, and sweeteners such as Splenda or Stevia. Keep an eye out for an excess of fructose from organic products too. If you are attempting to lose fat, limit organic products to only a couple of servings a day, or replace with non-boring vegetables.

Go for green vegetables

Although it is generally claimed that Paleo is a 'non-vegetable-friendly' diet, this is really not the case. Paleo restricts you mostly on starchy vegetables such as potatoes and corn. You can still incorporate green veggies such as spinach, cabbage and beans in Paleo, as that will improve your meal's nutrition content with iron, magnesium, lots of vitamins and fiber.

Avoid vegetable and seed oils

I know this can be difficult if you like eating out in restaurants, yet for home cooking—replace all seed oils with fat, ghee or coconut oil.

Stay away from most dairy items

Although the occasional use of full fat dairy products, such as unsweetened whip cream or Greek yogurt, won't necessarily hurt you (that is, if you aren't lactose intolerant), it's imperative that you stay away from all low fat and prepared types of dairy, such as skim or low fat yogurt.

Section B: The Many Paleo Benefits

Chapter 4: Weighing the Pros and Cons

According to health experts, food has advanced and changed more quickly than the human body, which hasn't adjusted to meet the needs of the normal human body processes. The outcome: Cellular aggravation and an increased chance of chronic diseases. In any case, many health issues connected with an average Western diet can probably be alleviated when a person returns to a more natural way of eating.

Here are the many amazing aspects of the Paleo diet that show the benefits for better health and wellbeing.

The Pros of Paleo

The Paleo diet is rich in soluble fiber, antioxidant vitamins, phytochemicals, omega-3 unsaturated fats, monounsaturated fat, and low-glycemic carbohydrates. Furthermore, it is actually gluten free and low in sugars, trans fats, salt, and high-glycemic carbohydrates. The diet makes exploring the universe of food and nutrition simple since there are no restrictions of eating less, counting calories, or guessing accurate serving sizes. Foods that individuals will probably indulge in, for example, a rich caramel chocolate brownie, are totally beyond reach. In this manner, the health benefits, increased energy levels, and general feeling of improved wellbeing might be less due to eating these foods and more due to removing the unhealthy foods from your diet.

Weight Loss

Paleo is more like a high-fat diet when it comes to the aspect of weight loss from eating caveman or ancestral types of foods. Your diet will comprise mainly of proteins and fats, and less carbs. This means, all your energy will come from fats burning in the body and not carbs.

When you get energy more from fats and less from carbs, this makes you burn more stored fat in your body and less carbs are needed, leading to weight loss.

Increased and More Stable Energy

The reason why Paleo is better than all other carb diets is that you get all your energy from fats and you should know that **one gram of fat provides you 9.5cal energy while same amount of carb provides 4.5cal.** This clearly means that eating more healthy fats will therefore increase your energy levels and keep you active throughout the day.

Improved Sleep

Good sleep is always a sign of better metabolism and health. When you eat Paleo food, this clearly increases your metabolism and energy levels thus keeping you active throughout the day to do all the tasks that you have to complete. Meanwhile, you won't feel tired or dizzy for a single moment while doing so. After a whole day, when you go to sleep, you will have a healthy 6 to 8 hours sleep that surely signifies a good health status and body metabolism.

Clearer Skin and hHealthier Hair

As you might know, the condition of your skin and hair are a great way for people to determine your age. When you have fresh, clean, healthy skin and hair, this makes you look healthy and youthful. Being on paleo provides all essential vitamins and proteins especially rich **keratin,** an essential protein for both skin and hair, thus keeping you looking healthy and young.

Better Mental Health

Scientists have recently proved that the brain can work faster, better and clearer when the energy supplied to its tissues is mainly from good fats like omega-3 and eicosanoids found in fish oil and nuts, etc. This clearly means that the Paleo diet provides you with such necessary good fats to keep your brain functioning at its peak throughout the day, as compared to most modern diets.

Lowered Depression and Anxiety

When you feel more active and boosted that means your brain is getting more energy to work properly and excitably. Experts suggest that our ancestors had more levels of **serotonin** on average than a normal human of today's modern age. This clearly points out the only difference between the two which is diet and our ancestors were paleo eaters.

Better Muscular Fitness

In paleo, all you eat is pure proteins from fish, mutton, beef, eggs, etc. You might know that muscles are completely made up of proteins which keep the strength of your muscles. When you work out, you actually need more proteins afterwards to increase the muscular mass. Working on a paleo diet gives you a better result because of the more protein intake that is a main component in eating paleo foods. Hence, working out and eating paleo makes the best combination, resulting in a healthier and active life with good muscular integrity and fitness.

Lowered Risk of Heart Disease, Diabetes and Cancer

Paleo food keeps you on track by promoting heart-healthy foods and antihypertensive nutrition as it contains more good fats and less bad fats, such as cholesterol which can increase risks of heart failure, heart attack and stroke by producing plaque in your blood vessels.

Moreover, Paleo diet foods have fewer carbohydrates and the carbs you take in are completely good carbs, unlike sugars, such as glucose. Although you do take in glucose in a very small quantity for the blood cells and certain parts of brain which rely on them, but it guards against the development of diabetes.

The most important thing about Paleo foods is that it contains antioxidants and inhibitors that help your cells to keep functioning properly while multiplying in a normal and controlled manner, thus reducing the possibility of cancer.

Healthier Immune System

Paleo foods are rich in nutrients like vitamin K, vitamin A and other immune-friendly nutritional supplements, like iron and potassium. These help your immune system cells to work and function more efficiently. A better immune system means stronger defense from allergies, diseases and other harmful issues. Eating Paleo keeps you from getting ill more than you should and keeps your immune system healthy and functioning properly.

Reduced Allergies

Seasonal allergies are something that no one desires to have and can keep you away from work and studies when that time of year arrives. Sometimes allergies are not seasonal but are due to certain foods that are eaten. The Paleo diet consists of foods that are scientifically proven to keep your immune system healthy, thus preventing any sort of food poisoning issue or food allergies. This, in turn, keeps you fit and also prevents you from having to take any medicines that can damage your immune system.

Improved Respiratory System

Now the most important thing about Paleo is the antihistamine function of healthy fats and proteins. Eating more dairy products and products that contain more of additives causes more histamine to be secreted in your respiratory tract. This will cause more instances of inflammation, flu and, most importantly, asthma. Eating Paleo gives you more foods containing antihistamine and gives purely nutritional, healthy supplements.

The Cons of Paleo

Although there are a few drawbacks of being on Paleo, you can eventually overcome these if you are educated and smart about how and when to eat Paleo foods.

➢ Whole grains and vegetables, which are not allowed on primal diets, are a critical source of fiber and supplements, and additionally an environmentally friendly source of plant-based protein.

➢ Paleo can be too hard for some individuals to maintain over a long period of time, which can prompt yo-yo dieting and poor general health.

➢ The substantial dependence on meat, which can be attributed to the Paleo diet, has over and over been connected to an increased potential of disease and can also be a burden on the earth's environment.

➢ Weight loss from restrictive diets is difficult to keep up over time; weight will be gained back if any "forbidden" foods are re-introduced into the diet.

➢ Extensive use of coconut oil and other coconut products, which are mainly imported, can leave a large food-related carbon footprint.

Section C: The Warm-Up

Chapter 5: Getting Motivated and Ready For Paleo

One of the biggest questions you may be asking yourself is how to keep your head up and stay motivated to take on the Paleo or primal diet for a lifetime or for a great amount of your life. It may take months for your to fully convert your diet into the Paleo diet category.

The main reason for lack of motivation on the Paleo diet is that you have spent your entire life developing the bad habit of eating the tasty, but unhealthy commercial foods, and now, all of a sudden, you have to give them up.

If you want motivation and a head start to stay on the diet for a longer time, this section of the book will give you the perfect outline for how you can do that.

Writing Your Goals

Take a small piece of paper and write each and every reason you want to adopt the Paleo life. Writing by hand on paper works best since it is slower, more physical and helps you think clearly and deeply. Therefore, writing on paper is more enjoyable and motivational than other options, like making notes in your phone or laptop.

So, begin right now to record each possible reason that you can think of to become Paleo. Try not to be too hard on yourself.

Best Reasons for Paleo

- ✓ You will look better.
- ✓ You will feel more accomplished in terms of improving your health.
- ✓ You will feel better physically, mentally and emotionally.
- ✓ You will be more content when you look in the mirror.

- ✓ You will be more confident.

- ✓ You will have more success in life.

- ✓ You will be able to beat depression and anxiety.

- ✓ You will have less uneasiness.

- ✓ You will have a higher quality of life.

- ✓ You will have the capacity to motivate and lead others.

- ✓ You will have more energy.

- ✓ You will have more courage.

- ✓ You will feel more in control.

- ✓ You will utilize your time better.

- ✓ You will have the capacity to play with your children.

- ✓ You will get off many medicines.

- ✓ You will have a healthier family.

- ✓ You will be more patient with others.

Weight Loss

This is one of the biggest and most motivational aspects of the Paleo diet and is the main reason why most people choose a Paleo lifestyle. Why should you choose Paleo to lose weight? The answer is very simple:

- ➤ Paleo keeps you full, thus preventing you from overeating.

- ➤ More healthy fats and less carbs gives your tummy a feeling of fullness.

- ➤ Proteins keep you motivated to exercise and burn more calories.

➢ Paleo inhibits the storage of extra fat in the body, hence keeping you slim and healthy.

Chapter 6: Pantry Makeover Time

Your kitchen cupboard or pantry is what clearly demonstrates which diet are you on. If you eat more commercial foods, and your pantry is full of food items that are technically not good for a better, Paleo diet, then you need to clean it all out. When you are about to begin the Paleo diet, you will have to eat fresh and healthy without any industrial food additives.

Cleaning Up the Mess

The most important thing to do before starting a Paleo diet is to get rid of factory packaged foods which contain many added chemicals. These actually include most of the dairy products on the market.

Before you get started, throw out all the foods in your fridge and pantry that you will not be eating on the Paleo diet. If you only have healthy options to choose from when you get hungry, then chances are you will make a healthy choice and stay on track.

Food items that are too expensive to simply throw out, like honey or cashews can be given away or kept for someone else in your home to eat.

Restocking

After cleaning out the foods that are not in keeping with starting a Paleo diet program, it is finally time to restock your pantry and kitchen with foods that are necessary. First, learn more about Paleo foods and the characteristics of good, Paleo foods. When trying to decide what foods to buy, always think about the main ingredients of that particular natural food by roughly estimating the total amount of healthy fats, bad fats, carbs, proteins, vitamins and other necessary minerals.

Opt for foods that provide more of the healthy fats and carbs, for your nutritional intake. Choose fats that are rich in omega-3's rather than trans fats or omega-6 fats. Proteins are also a necessary part of the diet, especially if you are thinking of hitting the gym during the dieting days.

Use your phone to search for nutritional values of any food item you want to buy but have no idea what it might contain.

Refreshing Your Pantry and Kitchen Every Week

One of the most important aspects of eating Paleo foods is eating them as fresh as possible. Therefore you need to refresh your stock often. This includes mainly meats and fleshy foods.

Similarly, fruits and vegetables should be refreshed every 2 or 3 days at most, as they can rot very quickly and become dangerously unhealthy if consumed.

When shopping for fish, consider that those with reddish gills are fresh, while those with no coloration in the gills are not fresh. However, unlike mutton and beef, you can buy an entire week's worth of fish at one time. You can also buy fish, mutton, and beef in bulk and stock it up in your freezer for the whole diet plan.

Dry fruits can be bought all at once and kept in the pantry, as they never expire. Meanwhile eggs should be replaced with meat. Keep 10-12 eggs maximum per week and try to divide them between breakfast or snacks by eating one or two each day.

Chapter 7: Essential Kitchen Ingredients

Having an excellent understanding of the foods you can eat while on Paleo will help you plan your daily meals. Always remember to keep things straightforward while setting up your meal plan. By keeping your food items simple and straightforward, your diet will remain free from the chemicals and food additives that are contained in commercially packaged food items.

In view of that, here is a rundown of foods you should choose from the store to kick off your Paleo lifestyle!

Paleo Meats

This is a list of the meats permitted on the Paleo eating regimen. All meats are "Paleo" by definition. Obviously, you'll need to avoid prepared meats and meats that are high in fat (meats such as spam, hot dogs, and other low-quality meats). Here's the full rundown of the Paleo meats.

- Turkey
- Chicken
- Steak
- Ground Beef
- Lobster
- Buffalo
- Rabbit
- Goat
- Elk
- Quail
- Ostrich

Paleo Fish

Fish are unquestionably on the Paleo diet and they're crammed with good stuff such as omega-3s. Here are some amazing options:

- Salmon
- Bass
- Tuna
- Sardines
- Trout
- Shark
- Walleye

Paleo Seafood

Check out all the different seafood you can eat on the Paleo diet.

- Crabs
- Crawfish
- Shrimps
- Lobster
- Oyster

Paleo Vegetables

Most vegetables are Paleo, however you should be careful here. Vegetables with high starch content, for example, potatoes and squashes, have a tendency to have low nutritional quality. While they're not terrible for you, they're not generally that great for you either.

- Asparagus
- Avocado

- Broccoli

- Spinach

- Carrots

- Celery

- Parsley

- Onions

- Cabbage

- Zucchini

Paleo Oils and Fats

Paleo opposes the mainstream thinking, **fat doesn't make you fat; carbs do**. Common oils and fats are your body's most important and effective source of providing you with high energy levels. So it's best to give your body what it's requesting. The following is a portion of the best sorts of Paleo oils and fats that you can give your body if you need some extra energy.

- Coconut oil

- Olive oil

- Macadamia oil

- Avocado oil

- Grass-fed butter

Paleo Nuts and Fruits

- Almonds

- Pecans

- Pine Nuts

- Pumpkin seeds

- Walnuts
- Apple
- Lemon
- Strawberries
- Watermelon
- Lime
- Raspberries
- Grapes
- Peaches
- Plums
- Mango
- Lychee
- Oranges
- Bananas
- Papaya

Chapter 8: Good vs. Bad Carbohydrates, Fats & Oils

Carbohydrates and fats are both essential nutrients of our life and we simply cannot live without them, as most of the body systems require them to work properly. Both fats and carbohydrates also make up the main basic nutritional supplements for humans.

But you should keep a check on the type of fats and carbohydrates you consume if you are eating for better health. Keeping a list of good and bad fats and carbs on the Paleo diet is essential. Make sure to eat only healthy carbs and fats that will work with your body instead of the bad carbs and fats that will slowly and gradually play havoc on your well-being.

You must have the proper knowledge about carbs and fats before selecting food items to include in your diet.

Good vs. Bad Carbs

In the past few years, the notoriety of carbohydrates has grown tremendously. Carbs have been touted as the dreaded food in fad diets. However, a few carbs have been promoted as a refreshing supplement connected with lowering the risk of chronic diseases.

So which is it? Are carbs good or bad? The short answer is that they are both.

Fortunately, it's simple to separate the good from the bad.

- You can profit from good carbs by picking carbohydrates loaded with fiber. These carbs get absorbed gradually into our bodies, without causing a spike in glucose levels. These good carbs include whole grains, vegetables, natural products, and beans, etc.

- Stay away from bad carbs. Bad carbs, which are refined and processed carbs, are bad for your body and can strip away healthy fiber. These bad carbs include such foods as white bread and white rice, etc.

Good Carbs Are:

- ➢ Lower in calories , which means we can eat them and feel more satisfied, yet not stress over going overboard on calories.

- ➢ High in a wide variety of supplements.

- ➢ Do not contain refined sugars and refined grains. In America, refined sugars, like corn syrup, now make up more than 20% of the calories we eat every day. That is a major issue in light of the fact that human bodies have advanced over hundreds and hundreds of years to metabolize bad carbohydrates. We're conditioned to handle them. We're ignorant regarding high fructose corn syrup. Daily, large amounts of sugar in our bloodstream are directly linked to our current epidemics of obesity and type 2 diabetes.

- ➢ High in fiber, which lowers glucose and insulin levels as well as LDL, bad cholesterol. Fiber-rich foods also offer you fewer calories so you can shed pounds more quickly. A high-fiber diet also counteracts constipation, hemorrhoids, and certain tumors. Americans normally consume only 12 to 15 grams of fiber a day. Nutrition experts say we should be getting no less than 35 to 50 fiber grams each day.

- ➢ Low in sodium.

- ➢ Low in saturated fat.

- ➢ Low (typically zero) cholesterol, and no trans fats.

Bad Carbs are

- ➢ High in calories. (Only a few bites of an energy bar, and you've consumed a lot of calories.)

- High in refined sugars (whether white sugar, corn syrup, or supposed "natural" sugars like honey and fruit juices).

- High in refined grains such as white flour.

- Low in vitamins.

- Low in fiber.

- High in sodium.

Good vs. Bad Fats

Fat is as key to your diet as protein and carbohydrates are, providing you with necessary energy. Dietary fat, which comes from the food you eat, is crucial to the absorption of fat-soluble vitamins, which includes vitamins A, D, K and E. Vitamins are essential, which means fats are essential, too. Without an adequate amount of fat in your diet, your body is unable to effectively absorb the fat-soluble vitamins that are essential to your health. However, that's not a free pass to consume a dozen donuts: The types of fat you eat matter...a lot.

All fats contain a mixture of saturated and unsaturated fatty acids but choosing foods which contain higher amounts of unsaturated "good" fat, and less saturated "bad" fat, is preferable.

Good Fats Are

Monounsaturated fat and polyunsaturated fat are viewed as more "heart-healthy" fats. These fats can have a beneficial effect on your heart when eaten in moderation. Foods that fundamentally contain these more advantageous fats have a tendency to be liquid when they're at room temperature.

Monounsaturated Fat

Studies show that eating foods rich in monounsaturated fatty acids improves blood cholesterol levels, which can decrease your risk of heart disease. These foods include:

- nuts (almonds, cashews, peanuts, pecans)

- vegetable oils (olive oil, canola oil, shelled nut oil)

- nutty spread and almond margarine

- avocado

Polyunsaturated Fat

This is a type of fat found mostly in plant-based foods and oils. Evidence shows that eating foods rich in polyunsaturated fatty acids improves blood cholesterol levels, which can decrease your risk of heart disease. These fatty acids may also help decrease the risk of type 2 diabetes.

One type of polyunsaturated fat is made up of mainly omega-3 fatty acids and may be especially beneficial to your heart. Omega-3, found in some types of fatty fish, appears to decrease the risk of coronary artery disease. There are also plant sources of omega-3 fatty acids. The following greasy fish contain omega-3 unsaturated fats:

- salmon

- herring

- sardines

- trout

You can also find omega-3s in flaxseed, walnuts, and canola oil, although these contain a less dynamic type of the fat than fish do.

Apart from omega-3 unsaturated fats, you can find polyunsaturated fat in the following foods, which contain omega-6 unsaturated fats:

- tofu

- cooked soy beans and soy nut margarine

- walnuts

- seeds (sunflower seeds, pumpkin seeds, sesame seeds)

- vegetable oils (corn oil, safflower oil, sesame oil, soybean oil, sunflower oil)

- margarine (fluid or tub)

Bad Fats Are

Two kinds of bad fats — saturated fat and trans fat — have been identified as potentially harmful to your heart. A large portion of the foods that contain these sorts of fats are solid at room temperature, for example:

- butter

- margarine

- shortening

- meat or pork fat

Both saturated fat and trans fat should be eliminated from your diet completely or eaten sparingly.

Saturated Fat

Saturated fat is animal- based, and is found in high-fat meats and dairy items. Some foods containing saturated fats include:

- greasy cuts of meat, pork, and sheep

- dark chicken meat and chicken skin

- high fat dairy foods (whole milk, margarine, cheddar, sour cream, frozen yogurt)

- tropical oils (coconut oil, palm oil, cocoa butter)

- lard

Trans Fat

Another way to say "trans unsaturated fats," trans fat is found in foods that contain mostly hydrogenated vegetable oils. These are the worse kind of fats for you. You may find trans-fat in:

- Deep fried foods (French fries, doughnuts, pan fried quick foods)

- margarine (stick and tub)

- vegetable shortening

- prepackaged foods (treats, cakes, pies, cookies)

- Snacks that you can eat at any time (wafers, microwave popcorn, etc.)

Like saturated fat, trans fat can raise LDL cholesterol, also known as "bad" cholesterol. Trans fat can also suppress high-density lipoprotein (HDL) levels, or "good" cholesterol. Trans fats, therefore, can raise your risk of heart disease three times higher than saturated fat intake.

Section D: Proper Meal Plan

Chapter 9: 21 Day Meal Plan

Now comes the most important part of this eBook, creating Paleo-friendly meals that you can stick to, while avoiding others. This diet plan is comprised of 21-days with three meals each day for breakfast, lunch and dinner. Remember, you can modify this plan according to your liking, but do not change the main concept If you wish to get the most benefit from it.

Week 1

Monday

Breakfast – Sausage and cucumber salad (use cubed avocados, cucumbers and sun-dried tomatoes with a vinaigrette dressing).

Lunch - Small plate of mixed greens: opt for a grilled fillet of salmon with mixed greens (including sautéed spinach, cabbage and boiled potato cubes), oil and vinegar.

Dinner - Butterflied cooked chicken with steamed veggies (use red beans, tomatoes, broccoli and spinach).

Tuesday

Breakfast – Black coffee with two eggs scrambled.

Lunch - Serving of mixed greens with extra butterflied cooked chicken, dried cranberries, pecans, apple cuts, and vinaigrette

Dinner - Ham and Pineapple skewers with seared tomatoes (makes 2 servings; keep leftovers for snacks)

Wednesday

Breakfast - Fried Eggs with Smoked Salmon.

Lunch – Warm chicken lettuce wraps with mustard, mayonnaise, or your favorite toppings, e.g. BBQ sauce, Hollandaise, etc.

Dinner - Greek-style meatballs (makes 2 days; use extras for any other meal tomorrow) with cooked cauliflower.

Thursday

Breakfast – Breakfast Frittata, eggs as the base and add whatever you like (bacon, onion, tomatoes, spinach, red pepper etc)

Lunch - Leftover Greek-style meatballs on top of a large plate of mixed greens with almond pieces and balsamic vinaigrette.

Dinner – Chicken roasted with low-fat butter. Make a carrot and kale salad as a side dish with vinaigrette. (makes 2 days; leftovers for lunch tomorrow).

Friday

Breakfast - Egg and Vegetable Muffins (makes 2 days; leftovers for tomorrow)

Lunch - Remaining roasted chicken with low-fat butter

Dinner – Hamburger (with minced meat patty and mustard sauce) with Roasted Carrots and Mushrooms (makes 2 days; leftovers for lunch tomorrow)

Saturday

Breakfast - Remaining egg and vegetable muffins

Lunch – Remaining hamburger (with minced meat patty and mustard sauce) with Roasted Carrots and Mushrooms

Dinner - Garlic Roasted Cod (2 medium fillets with lemon and mayo sauce) with green beans

Sunday

Breakfast – Onions, mushrooms and spinach sautéed with bacon.

Lunch - Salad with canned salmon, mustard vinaigrette.

Dinner - Maple Braised Chuck Roast (makes 2 servings; leftovers for lunch tomorrow) with cooked zucchini

Week 2

Monday

Breakfast - Apple and Onion Scrambled eggs with some additional browned onions and mushrooms

Lunch - Remaining maple braised chuck roast

Dinner - Grilled fish with an easy tomato soup (use 2 blanched tomatoes, blend them, add in boiling chicken stock with generous seasoning)

Tuesday

Breakfast – Smoothie made with 1 cup frozen mixed berries, 1 cup fresh spinach, 1 cup coconut water, ½ cup coconut milk, plus a small amount of protein such as 3 slices of baked chicken

Lunch - Convenient salad: Dice an avocado with some salad greens, oil, and vinegar. Eat the salad with a simple grilled steak.

Dinner – Sunday roast – roasted free range chicken with lemon, mustard and rosemary, roasted carrots, fennel, whole garlic cloves and beetroot, steamed greens such as broccoli or green peas with mint and butter (makes 2, enough for lunch leftovers)

Wednesday

Breakfast - Breakfast stuffed peppers Roasted cauliflowers with grilled pork steak.

Lunch – Remaining Sunday roast

Dinner - Flame grilled chicken breast with zucchini (leave a large portion of the chicken for lunch tomorrow)

Thursday

Breakfast - Remaining breakfast stuffed peppers

Lunch - Remaining flame grilled chicken cubes on top of salad greens with vinaigrette

Dinner – Roasted cauliflowers with grilled pork steak (makes 2 servings; leftovers for lunch tomorrow)

Friday

Breakfast - Two semi soft-boiled eggs chopped over a bed of wilted spinach leaves with olive oil, lemon and garlic. Topped with ½ cup cherry tomatoes, ½ avocado, ¼ cup diced green onion and drizzled with lemon juice,

Lunch – Remaining roasted cauliflowers with grilled pork steak.

Dinner – Grilled beef (makes 2 servings; leftovers for breakfast tomorrow) with grilled beets and sweet potatoes. Broil a double batch of vegetables so you have some for lunch tomorrow.

Saturday

Breakfast - Egg scrambled with sautéed onion, can add extras like red peppers, bacon tomatoes, served with a side salad of avocado, coriander, lime juice and olive oil.

Lunch - Remaining beef steak served over sautéed spinach

Dinner – Seafood platter – 4-5 grilled prawns, 3-4 oysters, calamari, octopus or mussels with a side green salad

Sunday

Breakfast - Cherry Tomato and Basil Quiche with additional sautéed onions

Lunch – Grilled Chicken drumsticks with honey and mustard, served with a kale and raspberry salad.

Dinner – 200g grass fed beef steak marinated for an hour or 2 with rosemary, garlic, lemon juice, sea salt and pepper, grilled to medium rare in ghee or coconut oil. Serve it with a grilled Portobello mushroom and 2 cups of slaw salad made with shredded red cabbage, carrot, Spanish onion, parsley and dressing with lemon juice, 1 tablespoon mayonnaise and 1 tablespoon extra-virgin olive oil.

Week3

Monday

Breakfast - 2 eggs and bacon (cook the eggs how you like them)

Lunch – 2 lamb sausages with grilled asparagus and a side of spinach salad with red peppers, sesame seeds and tahini, lemon juice and extra-virgin olive oil dressing. Add a dollop of Dijon or wholegrain mustard on the side.

Dinner – Paleo Fried rice (use cauliflower rice as the base, add prawns, onions, red bell peppers, peas) will have enough leftovers for lunch

Tuesday

Breakfast – Onions, mushrooms, and spinach fried up with bacon or sausages.

Lunch - Tuna salad with an apple

Dinner – Salmon fillet encrusted with almonds (add minced almonds, garlic, dill, lemon zest, honey, Dijon mustard) serve with greens. (make enough for leftovers)

Wednesday

Breakfast - Fresh strawberries and bananas

Lunch - Salmon fillet encrusted with almonds leftovers

Dinner - Grilled steak and mashed cauliflower

Thursday

Breakfast - Green smoothie (kale and kiwi) add to a blender with fruit and some ice.

Lunch – Jalapeno poppers (see recipe section)

Dinner – mushroom and baby corn spaghetti topped with a slice of mozzarella cheese (use zucchini spaghetti)

Friday

Breakfast – 2 fried eggs with salad. Combine fresh baby spinach, peppers, onion, carrots, tomato, celery, avocado, broccoli or any of your favorite vegetables.

Lunch - BLT Salad with Prawns & Avocado. Make a salad of lettuce, cherry tomatoes, capsicum/bell peppers, avocado, dress with combined Dijon mustard, mayonnaise and lime juice) add prawns and bacon.

Dinner – Duck with roasted vegetables (see recipe section)

Saturday

Breakfast - Paleo flapjacks with strawberries or blueberries

Lunch - Caramelised Onion, tomato & Ham Omelette Roll.

Dinner – Marjoram & Tomato Chicken Skewers (Combine dried marjoram with chopped garlic, tomato paste, olive oil, and rub over chicken tenderloins skewers) serve with dressed green salad leaves

Sunday

Breakfast – Ham and butternut squash hash (see recipes section)

Lunch - Paleo Sushi with Salmon (use telegraph cucumber cut into rounds, scoop the inside outs to form a hole), add salmon fillet, avocado, red onion mixture

Dinner – Shepherd's Pie with Cauliflower topping.

38

Chapter 10: Recipes for Success

Breakfast

Prosciutto-Wrapped Mini Frittata Muffins

Total Serves – 2

Preparation Time – 25 minutes

Ingredients

- Fat (coconut oil, ghee, etc.) – Four tbsp.

- Onion, finely diced- Half medium sized

- Garlic, minced – Three cloves

- Cremini mushrooms, thinly sliced- half pound

- Frozen spinach, thawed and squeezed dry – half pound

- eggs – Eight large

- coconut milk – Quarter of a cup

- coconut flour – Two tbsp.

- cherry tomatoes, halved – One cup

- Kosher salt

- Freshly ground pepper

- A regular 12 cup muffin tin

Nutritional Information

- 861 calories

- 123g fat (2 g saturated)

- 170 g carbs (0.9 g fiber)

- 21.5 g sugars

- 164 g protein

Instructions

1. Preheat oven at 380 degrees.

2. Heat coconut oil and onion in pan until melted. Add garlic and mushroom to it and cook further. Then add salt and pepper and cool at room temperature.

3. Beat the eggs in a large bowl with coconut milk, coconut flour, salt, and pepper until well-mixed.

4. Fill the muffin tins with it and bake oven for 20 minutes.

Citrus and Avocado Salad

Total Serves – 2

Preparation Time – 16 minutes

Ingredients

- oranges, peeled and sliced -Five

- oranges, peeled and sliced - Two

- fennel bulb, very thinly sliced - Half

- avocado, sliced - One

- scallion, very thinly sliced - One

- extra-virgin olive oil – One third of a cup

- apple cider vinegar – Two tbsp.

- honey (optional) - 1 tbsp.

- Fresh dill

- Sea salt and freshly ground black pepper

Nutritional Information

- 261 calories

- 0 g fat (0 g saturated)

- 50 g carbs (0.9 g fiber)

- 31.5 g sugars

- 14 g protein

Instructions

1. On a serving plate, stack all the slices of oranges in a layer and top with the avocado and fennel.

2. In a small bowl, mix and blend the olive oil, vinegar, honey (if using), and salt and pepper to taste.

3. Pour the dressing over the salad with scallions and fresh dill.

Snacks

Chocolate-Coconut Bites

Total Serves – 2

Preparation Time – 15 minutes

Ingredients

- coconut oil, melted – half cup

- raw cocoa powder – half cup

- Raw honey or maple syrup – Two tbsp.

- pure vanilla extract – Half tbsp.

- Toppings of your own choice

- Sea salt – as needed

Nutritional Information
• 370 calories
• 21 g fat (6 g saturated)
• 62 g carbs (7.9 g fiber)
• 35.5 g sugars
• 40 g protein

Instructions

1. In a dish, whisk the cocoa powder with the softened coconut oil until smooth.

2. Combine all the remaining ingredients, stir until smooth, and season with a pinch of salt.

3. Empty the liquid into your choice of pans or muffin tins, and pour ingredients in.

4. Chill for 15 to 20 minutes.

5. Take it out of the fridge a few minutes before serving.

Coconut Date Balls

Total Serves – 4

Preparation Time – 20 minutes

Ingredients

- dates, finely chopped – half cup

- eggs, beaten -Two

- raw honey – half cup

- Vanilla extract – One tbsp.

- ghee – Quarter of a cup

- mixed nuts, finely chopped – Two cups

- coconut flakes – One cup

- sea salt – One teaspoon

Nutritional Information
• 524 calories
• 41 g fat (11 g saturated)
• 31g carbs (8.9 g fiber)
• 43 g sugars
• 71 g protein

Instructions

1. Mix the eggs, ghee, craw honey, and dates in a medium pan and cook over medium heat.

2. Heat everything to the point of boiling, blending once in a while, for 3 to 5 minutes.

3. Remove it from the heat, blend in the vanilla, and add the sea salt.

4. Blend in the chopped nuts and mix until well combined.

5. Roll the mixture into little balls.

6. Roll each ball in the coconut flakes.

7. Refrigerate until firm.

Lunch

Jalapeno Poppers

Serves – 2

Time – 30 minutes

Ingredients:

1. 6 Bacon Slices

2. Cream Cheese (4 Oz.)

3. Cheddar Cheese shredded (4 Oz.)

4. Jalapeno slices (1.5 Oz.)

5. 2 eggs

6. Almond flour (4 tablespoons)

7. Parmesan Cheese (2 tablespoons)

8. Water (1 tablespoon

Nutrition Information
• Serving size: 5 Balls
• Calories: 387
• Fat: 33
• Carbohydrates: 4
• Fiber: 1
• Protein: 22

Instructions:

1. Cook the bacon thoroughly and crumble.

2. Chop up all the slices of Jalapeno

3. Mix the cream cheese, cheddar cheese, Jalapeno slices and prepared bacon

4. Make 20 balls of this mixture and put them in refrigerator

5. Meanwhile, make the batter by adding the almond flour to the whisked eggs and Parmesan cheese

6. Coat the balls with the batter and put them in fridge again

7. Fry the balls till they are golden brown

Portobello Mushroom Paleo Taco

Total Serves – 2

Preparation Time – 23 minutes

Ingredients

- Mushrooms – four medium

- large onion (chopped) – Half or quarter

- ground beef – Half kg

- red chili pepper (diced) - One

- garlic - One clove

- ghee – Half tbsp.

- salt to taste

- green onions (finely chopped) - Two

- cherry tomatoes (sliced) – Half cup

- olives (sliced) – Half cup

Instructions

Nutritional Information
• 415 calories
• 31 g fat (9 g saturated)
• 25 g carbs (5.9 g fiber)
• 21 g sugars
• 102 g protein

1. Preheat oven to 450 F.

2. In a large skillet or medium pot, cook onions in ghee over medium heat until soft.

3. Remove stems and spoon out mushroom inner parts. Dice finely and add to onions.

4. Add ground meat and diced peppers. Once seared, add taco flavoring and salt (if needed).

5. Cook the mushrooms for 8 minutes on one side and 8 minutes on the other side, when it is brown on both sides, heat for an additional 10 minutes to give it a firm texture.

6. Spoon ground beef into mushrooms, followed by tomatoes, olives, green onions, and garlic.

Dinner

Baked Salmon with Lemon and Thyme

Total Serves – 2

Preparation Time – 23 minutes

Ingredients

- Salmon – Half kg

- lemon, sliced thin - One

- Capers – One tbsp.

- Salt and freshly ground pepper

- Fresh thyme – One tbsp.

Nutritional Information

- 456 calories

- 56 g fat (15g saturated)

- 27 g carbs (7 g fiber)

- 14 g sugars

- 77 g protein

- Olive oil - for drizzling

Instructions

1. Line a rimmed baking sheet with wax paper and place salmon, skin side down, on the prepared baking sheet. Liberally season salmon with salt and pepper. Coat the salmon well and with lemon juice and thyme.

2. Place baking sheet in a cold oven, then turn the heatto 400 degrees F. Bake for 25 minutes. Serve promptly.

Duck with Roasted Vegetables

Total Serves – 4

Preparation Time – 40 minutes

Ingredients

- Duck – One medium

- Oranges – Two or three

- Rosemary – One bunch

- Carrots – Five or six

- Parsnips -Six

- Leeks - Three

- garlic, crushed – Three cloves

- Freshly ground black pepper

Nutritional Information
• 600 calories
• 76 g fat (22g saturated)
• 47 g carbs (11 g fiber)
• 16 g sugars
• 156 g protein

Instructions

1. Crush the garlic in a garlic press. Cut the carrots and parsnips into small pieces. Cut the leeks into 1-inch rounds.

2. Blend all of the vegetables with the crushed garlic and spread this mixture on the bottom of a broiling dish.

3. Cut the oranges into quarters. Stuff the orange pieces and the rosemary into the pit of the duck.

4. Sprinkle the duck with some ground black pepper.

5. Place the duck on top of the cooked vegetables.

6. Place the dish into the oven at 375F. Bake for about 45 minutes. Remove the dish from the oven and, using a baster, spread the juices over the duck and the vegetables. This keeps them from drying out.

7. Season occasionally until the duck is completely cooked. Maximum cooking time should be about 2.5 hours.

Other recipes to know

Butterflied cooked chicken

Total Serves – 2

Preparation Time – 45 minutes

Ingredients

- Chicken – One whole

- Paleo fat/oil – 3 tbsp.

- Rosemary – 3tbsp.

- Onions - Two

Nutritional Information

- 550 calories

- 56 g fat (22g saturated)

- 34 g carbs (11 g fiber)

- 14 g sugars

- 179 g protein

- Carrots - four

- Bell peppers - four

- Lemons - Two

- Sea salt and freshly ground black pepper to taste

Instructions

1. Preheat oven to 400 degrees. Cut the chicken into average pieces and set aside the backbone (do not use the backbone in recipe)

2. In a bowl, combine the fat, and rosemary.

3. Rub the chicken with rosemary and season the chicken to taste with salt and pepper.

4. Line a large dish with aluminum foil.

5. Place the chicken on top of the cooked vegetables.

6. Place the dish in the oven and cook for 45 minutes or until a meat thermometer reads 175 F in the thickest part of the breast.

7. Remove chicken from oven, squeeze some lemon juice over it, and serve.

Greek styled meatballs

Total Serves –4

Preparation Time – 25 minutes

Ingredients

- Ground beef – One kg

- Egg – One (beaten)

- Garlic cloves - Two

- Fresh parsley – Half cup

- Tomato paste – 2 tbsp.

- Oregano – half tbsp.

- Dried mint – One tbsp.

Nutritional Information

- 350 calories

- 66 g fat (18g saturated)

- 34.5 g carbs (10 g fiber)

- 7 g sugars

- 200 g protein

- Sea salt and freshly ground black pepper

Instructions

1. Preheat oven to 370 degrees.

2. In a bowl, mix an egg, parsley, garlic, ground beef, mint and season with salt and pepper.

3. Form equally shaped and sized meatballs.

4. Bake for 25 to 30 minutes in oven.

Ham and Butternut Squash Hash

Total Serves –4

Preparation Time – 25 minutes

Ingredients

- Butternut squash – One

- Pre-cooked ham, cubed – Two cups

Nutritional Information

- 460 calories

- 45 g fat (18g saturated)

- 45.6 g carbs (10 g fiber)

- 11 g sugars

- 234 g protein

- Leek - One

- Apple – One (green)

- Onion – One

- Garlic clove - Two

- Paprika – One tbsp.

- Ground cinnamon – One tsp.

- Cooking fat – as needed

- Sea salt and freshly ground black pepper

Instructions

1. Melt cooking fat over heat in skillet.

2. Cook the garlic and onion for 3 or 4 minutes.

3. Add the butternut squash and sliced leek, and cook until soft and tender (up to 10 min).

4. Season with all leftover ingredients.

5. Cook for 3 more minutes and serve.

Egg and Vegetable Muffins

Total Serves –2

Preparation Time – 18 minutes

Ingredients

- Eggs (beaten) - eight

- bell peppers - Two

- onion - One

- fresh mushrooms – eight to ten

- baby spinach – Two cups

- garlic cloves- Two

- Cooking fat – as needed

- Sea salt and freshly ground black pepper;

Nutritional Information
- 270calories
- 34 g fat (11g saturated)
- 35g carbs (12 g fiber)
- 14g sugars
- 240 g protein

Instructions

1. Preheat the oven to 380F.

2. Melt the cooking fat in skillet for a few minutes over medium heat. Cook the onion, bell peppers for about five minutes.

3. Add the mushroom and spinach and cook for five more minutes.

4. Whisk the eggs together and add it to the mixture. Pour the mixture into muffin tins.

5. Place in oven and bake for 15 minutes.

Maple Braised Chuck Roast

Total Serves – 4 to 6

Preparation Time – 38 minutes

Ingredients

- beef chuck roast – Two kg

- large onions - Three

- chicken stock – Two cups

- Dijon mustard – One tbsp.

- Maple syrup – One tbsp.

- Balsamic vinegar – One tbsp.

- Paprika – One tsp.

- Kosher salt – One tsp.

- Freshly ground black pepper - to taste

- Fresh thyme - to garnish

Nutritional Information

- 345 calories

- 41 g fat (13.5g saturated)

- 41 g carbs (13 g fiber)

- 12 g sugars

- 236 g protein

Instructions

1. Pat the beef dry with paper towels and season generously with salt and pepper.

2. In a separate bowl, whisk the chicken stock, Dijon, balsamic vinegar, maple syrup, paprika, salt, and pepper until combined.

3. Pour the onions and pan juices into the bowl of the slow cooker.

4. Pour the cooking liquids into large saucepan and bring to a boil. Cook until the gravy is reduced to desired thickness.

5. Serve.

Cherry Tomato and Basil Quiche

Total Serves –2

Preparation Time – 15 minutes

Ingredients

- Eggs - four

- garlic clove – One minced

- fresh basil – One bunch

- cherry tomatoes – half cup

- almond cheese – Half cup

- Sea salt and freshly ground black pepper

Nutritional Information
• 342 calories
• 44 g fat (15g saturated)
• 36g carbs (11 g fiber)
• 13g sugars
• 276 g protein

Instructions

1. Preheat the oven to 370F

2. In a bowl, beat the eggs, almond cheese, fresh basil until well combined. Season with salt and pepper to taste.

3. Pour all this in a baking dish.

4. Place in oven and bake for 15 minutes.

Paleo Flapjacks with Strawberries or Blueberries

Total Serves – 2

Preparation Time – 25 minutes

Ingredients

- Ghee/coconut oil or butter – Hundred grams

- Honey – hundred grams

- Oats – 150 grams

- shredded coconut – fifty grams

- raisins – 50 grams

- cinnamon – two teaspoons

- Strawberries – topping

Nutritional Information

- 400 calories

- 45 g fat (16g saturated)

- 44g carbs (17 g fiber)

- 26g sugars

- 170 g protein

Instructions

1. Preheat the oven to 180F.

2. Line baking dish with baking paper.

3. Heat the ghee or coconut oil and honey in sauce pan till it boils.

4. Mix the oats, coconut, cinnamon and raisins in a bowl separately. Pour the mixture into the prepared baking dish and distribute it evenly.

5. Place in oven and bake for 20 minutes.

Section E: Bonus Chapter!

Chapter 11: 3 Drinks for Paleo that literally take 5 minutes

Raspberry Coconut Smoothie

Total Serves – 1

Preparation Time – 5 minutes

Ingredients

- Raspberries (frozen) – One cup

- Coconut Milk – Half cup

- Banana (medium sized) – One

- Coconut extract – Two teaspoons

- Chocolate syrups or fruits sprinkles – Optional

Nutritional Information
• 261 calories
• 0 g fat (0 g saturated)
• 50 g carbs (0.9 g fiber)
• 31.5 g sugars
• 14 g protein

Instructions

1. Put coconut milk, frozen banana slices and coconut milk to your blender. Blend for about 3 minutes.

2. Add frozen raspberries and keep on blending it until smooth.

3. Pour the smoothie in your serving glass, top with several raspberries and a bit of shredded coconut, and drink while chilled!

Skinny Almond Butter Banana Smoothie

Total Serves – 2

Preparation Time – 5 minutes

Ingredients

- Bananas – Two frozen

- vanilla almond milk (unsweetened) – One cup

- Vanilla – One teaspoon

- Almond butter – One tbsp.

- Chia seeds – One teaspoon

Nutritional Information

- 180 calories

- 7 g fat (0.7 g saturated)

- 30 g carbs (4 g fiber)

- 15 g sugars

- 4 g protein

Instructions

1. Put all ingredients in a blender and blend on high speed for about 60 seconds until smooth.

2. Serve and enjoy.

Brownie Batter Smoothie

Total Serves – 2

Preparation Time – 5 minutes

Ingredients

- almond milk – Two cups

- banana (frozen) - One

- dates (pitted) - Four

- Cocoa powder – Two tbsp.

- Coconut flakes – Two tbsp.

Instructions

1. Add all ingredients in blender.

2. Blend for two minutes or 90 seconds.

3. Serve and enjoy.

Nutritional Information

- 160 calories

- 5.5 g fat (1.6 g saturated)

- 34 g carbs (5.5 g fiber)

- 16.5 g sugars

- 10.5 g protein

Conclusion

Now that you've read the entire eBook, you must realize that the Paleo diet is not limited to your kitchen. In fact, it includes every aspect of your daily life and helps you live a healthy and active lifestyle. After all, this diet invariably relates to the crude diet of the Stone Age era, and helps us get the most nutrition in the most profitable and raw form.

It not only provides a way to lose weight and stay physically fit and good looking, but also provides many other health benefits that specifically target cardiovascular, nervous, digestive or respiratory systems. The Paleo diet also regulates the serotonin levels in your brain, thus boosting your mood throughout the day, and eleminating mood swings.

The main idea of Paleo is based on eating the right amount and kind of calories required for proper functioning of your body and giving up products sold commercially that have been bombarded with many chemicals and additives, especially dairy products. Also, the main concept of Paleo focuses on eating proper portions of carbs, fats and proteins as stated in this eBook. The Paleo diet, in short, takes you back to the Stone Age where all that the caveman ate was raw and fresh, with pure health benefits rather than the fad diets of the modern age.

Use this eBook as a Paleo guide for information about this diet, beginning with the basics, to information and recipes needed at the pro level, the benefits, tips and lifestyle modification plans. Remember to stick to your plan and follow it at least 2 weeks consecutively to see the results and adopt this diet as a complete lifestyle package. It is only then that Paleo will fully benefit you and your family. You are sure to love this positive change in life, and we hope you continue it lifelong.

Stay healthy and eat delicious!

Good luck!

Caroline

More books by Caroline

I've had a personally enriching experience writing this book and hope that it translates to you too. Remember that I am with you at every step of this journey and have your back at all times. Finally, if you liked this book, then make sure you read my other books too. I guarantee that you'll be equally pleased with the experience.

Nutribullet Recipe Book

Here, I give you in-depth knowledge on the diet that's taken the fitness world by storm- The Nutribullet Diet. The diet emphasises on healthy living while showing you ways to incorporate liquid diets into your lifestyle. In my book, I share with you first-hand experiences and hand-picked recipes, its certain to leave you with the best detox plan you've ever known. Designed for detoxification, weight loss and healthy living, my book is sure to leave you inspired for live. You can purchase my book by visiting: NutriBullet Recipe Book

Bonus FREE Report – A gift from me to you

"6 Proven Health Benefits of Apple Cider Vinegar"

A miracle ingredient whose benefits range from healing skin allergies, killing harmful gut-bacteria, aiding digestion, controlling diabetes, reducing bad cholesterol, promoting weight loss, treating dandruff to preventing cancer and heart ailments, Apple Cider Vinegar is a versatile food component that goes beyond being just a cupboard-ingredient. In my book, I share with you the nutritional facts and beneficial properties of this highly handy fermented liquid. You can download my report by visiting: www.Freevinegar.com

Well, what are you waiting for? Make sure you grab a copy now!

Caroline